KEEP FIT

Nester Kadzviti Murira

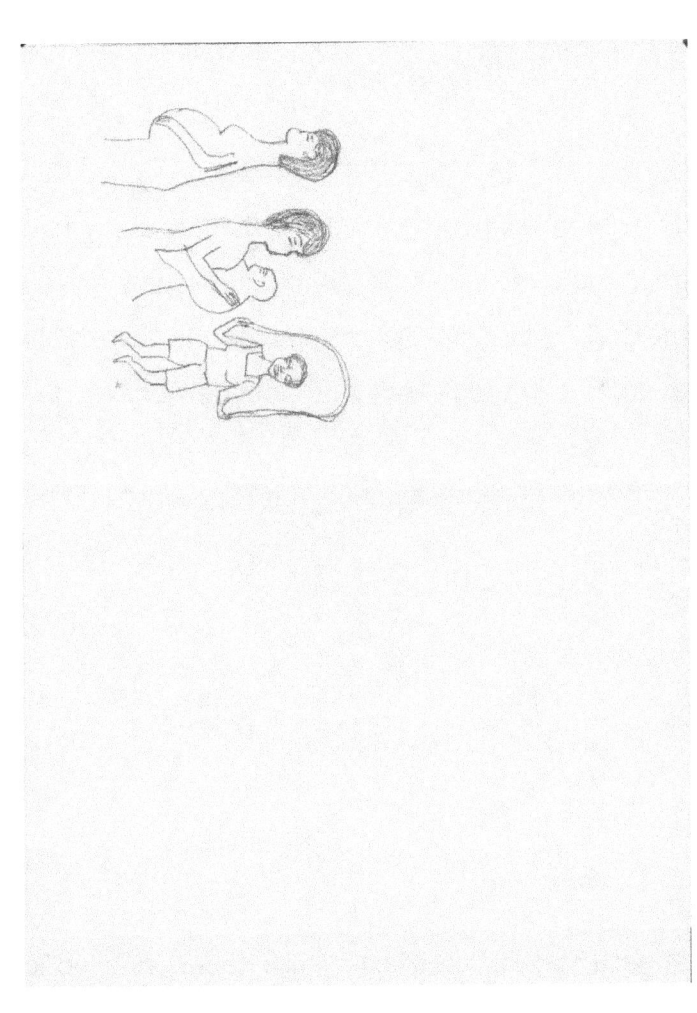

The information in this booklet is designed to keep your body as fit as possible as well as making you as comfortable as possible everyday, in pregnancy and post delivery.

At each stage of the woman's life, there are specific exercises a woman has to be aware of that focus on the bodily changes taking place during the specific times. Exercise requirements in the woman's life can be arranged to suit women in the period before pregnancy, in the first three months of pregnancy, second three months of pregnancy, third or final three months of pregnancy and the period after the birth of a child.

"Culture is obsessed with appearance. In some cultures, loss of weight is equated to self control. Bodily perfection is equated to moral perfection. Physical beauty is a result of hard work, ambition and self control. The overweight are what they are because they are lazy to do something about their weight and are self indulgent" (Lee, 1998).

Exercises throughout the lifeline are designed to suit the changes in body, the recovery after delivery, and maintaining good health and shape everyday. After having a baby, women must make an effort to return back to shape by shedding off the massive weight gained during pregnancy.

The Importance of Exercise

Exercise is important for **improvement of general physical fitness**.

As one exercises, stored fats and carbohydrates are burnt up and used as energy.

- Excess water and wastes from your body are lost through sweat.
- Exercise strengthens muscles improve shape, stable gait and good posture.
- Exercise in general is important for **movement of body joints** and prevents stiff joints and general aches and pains. Where there is limited joint movement or rigidity, exercise improves muscle and joint movement reducing the aches and pains.
- Exercise is important for the body to maintain **good body balance especially in pregnancy where one is carrying a gradually increasing body weight**.

- Activity **improves blood flow**, makes the heart to beat harder and faster pumping blood to all parts of the body.
- Through exercises, sagging smooth muscles are tightened, fluid sitting in wrong places in the body is moved and ankle swelling (oedema) reduced.
- The increase in the breathing rate during exercises **draws in more air to the lungs**, which expand to the maximum. The fresh air is passed onto the blood as the blood gives off carbon dioxide from muscle activity. The fresh blood prevents muscle cramps.
- **Exercise improves appetite.** In early pregnancy women generally may have loss of appetite for major groups of food that are essential in keeping the body healthy. With good regular exercise, a pregnant woman's appetite gradually improves.

- **Exercise improves sleep**. After walking for about twenty to thirty minutes, it is possible for one to enjoy a good nap later on in the day or a good night's sleep.
- In pregnancy, an early morning or evening walk over a stretch of a distance is encouraged to improve circulation of blood around the body.

Pregnancy and Exercise

Being pregnant exposes your body to physical challenges that are addressed in this booklet.

Exercises in pregnancy focuses on certain groups of muscles that may be particularly affected by pregnancy hormones.

- You must take care that you do not strain yourself. Any exercises that cause you significant pain and sweating should be avoided.
- You should however feel that the exercise you are engaged in makes a positive difference to how you feel. Your body or the group of muscles you are trying to tone or relax will feel positively different and you should feel good after the exercise.

The back/The spine

The spine or backbone extends from the neck to the pelvis. It supports all the structures of the body. It enables you to bend, balance when you walk or when you stretch to reach for things.

- You should therefore look after it well not just in pregnancy but everyday. The hormones of pregnancy soften the rubbery tissue **(cartilage)** between the spinal bones.
- As pregnancy advances, the weight of the pregnancy may cause one to alter her posture resulting in the back leaning backwards.
- One may experience backache especially over the lumbar spine region.

Care of the Back

Make a conscious effort to keep your back straight. Do not throw yourself backwards as you walk; this causes severe backache and bad posture.

Swing your arms as you walk to relax your joints and promote good flow of blood to your fingers.

- Sit on straight chairs with a firm back that supports your back to prevent it from sagging backwards.
- Put a small pillow or cushion behind the small of the back which is the part of the spine that is mostly affected by pregnancy and may cause you backache.
- Avoid bending or doubling up to perform household tasks or to pick items from the floor.
- Bend your knees with one leg forward to pick items or crouch just like the toddler does to pick items from the floor.
- Do not carry heavy objects in one arm, carry even loads in both arms
- Do not lift heavy items.
- Where possible, do as much of your domestic work while sitting

- Lye on your left side when you take a rest, use pillows and cushions to support your tummy or back to increase your comfort.
- Roll out of bed from one side; do not jump out of bed or lift your back to sit up before getting out of bed.
- Adopt comfortable sexual positions that do not cause backache such as:

  (i)Go on fours with your partner approaching from the back

  (ii)Lye on your side with your partner approaching from the rear

  (iii) Sit on your partner's lap

  (iv) Sit in an upright position on your partner while your partner lies on his back (see diagrams).

MASSAGE

Massage plays an important role in pregnancy. It is useful in:

- Moving body fluids from around the ankles and feet relieving swelling of ankles and feet.
- Massage relaxes and stimulates nerves, improves circulation thus relieving numbness, tense muscles, stress, dull aches and pains.
- Your partner, a physiotherapist and massage parlours can assist in providing gentle massage on different groups of muscles in your body.
- Your partner should therefore attend antenatal classes with you so that he is familiar with massaging.
- Massage requires that you are both relaxed and not in a hurry.

- The sitting position is most comfortable for massage in pregnancy as your partner is able to reach any part of the body to be massaged.

Foot and ankle massage

The legs bear the body weight as a pregnant mother stands or walks. Fluid collects around the ankles and feet due to the pressure of the growing baby weighing heavily on the blood vessels of the lower leg.

- Massage of the foot and ankle relieves tension and moves fluid from the feet upwards the leg towards the heart.
- Relief of foot and ankle swelling is more effective if you combine massage with elevating your feet on a foot stool or cushion when you sit.
- Soak feet in warm water, your partner can then wash them and oil them making circular movements with the palms and

gently making upward movements intended to encourage fluid to move up the leg towards the heart.

- Foot and ankle exercise helps to relax the joints and also move the body fluid reducing and preventing ankle oedema.
- Move the foot from the ankle in upwards and downwards movements up to ten times.

- Move the foot in circular movements ten times towards the left then towards the right side. Move the toes up and down ten times. Repeat these movements three times whenever you have an opportunity while you relax.

The Lower Leg Massage

The hormones of pregnancy relax the smooth muscles of the lower legs including the blood vessels.

As the blood vessels relax, there is reduced pressure to push blood back to the heart.

- The pressure of the growing baby on the blood vessels of the lower legs also slows down the flow of blood back to the heart.
- Blood pools in the relaxed veins of the lower legs which are forced to stretch out to hold blood causing the dark wavy veins that can be seen behind the legs (**varicose veins**).

- Varicose veins are ugly and can be painful. Some varicose veins can burst open becoming ugly wounds.
- It is best to engage in leg exercises and massage of the lower leg to improve blood circulation and prevent varicose veins.
- Massage of the lower leg is aimed at moving blood and other body fluids towards the heart where the blood is distributed to other parts of the body.
- Massage movements must therefore be upwards towards the heart using the palms and gently kneading the muscles with flat fingers. Do not squeeze the muscles.
- While seated in a firm chair, with feet flat on the floor, move your legs up and down in marching rhythm ten times.
- Move your legs in gentle kicking movement's one leg at a time ten times.

- If you have access to stairs then you can go up and down two stairs.
- Walking is one wonderful exercise that moves all the leg muscles, and encourages blood flow up and down the legs.
- Walking reduces tension in the pelvis, relaxes joints and encourages the baby to change position relieving pressure in the pelvis.

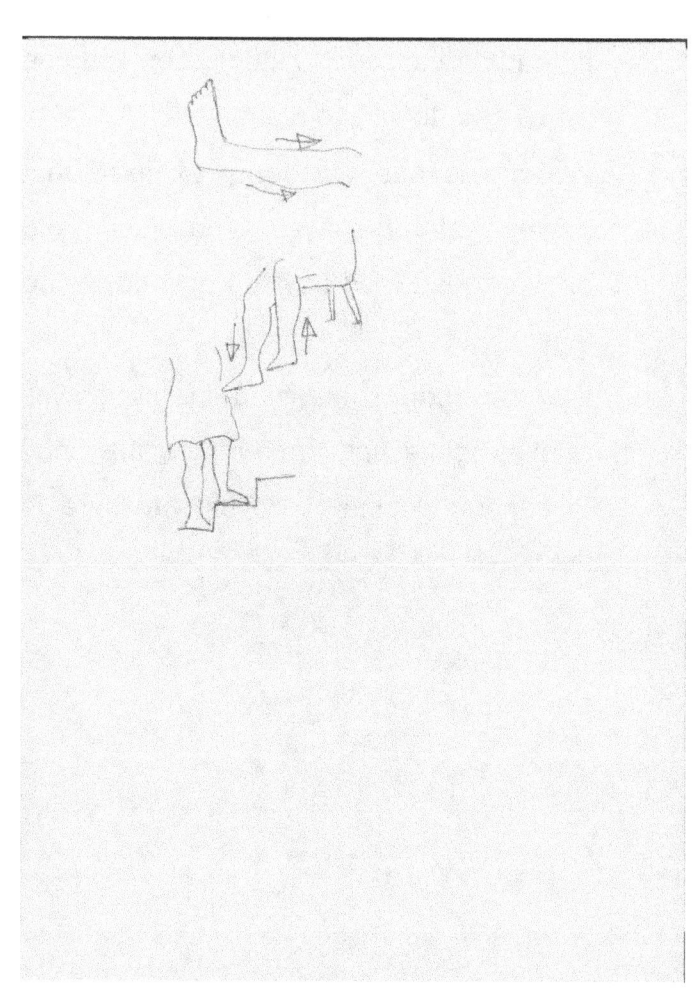

The Thighs

- Your thighs are affected by the hormones of pregnancy and the muscles become relaxed and flabby.
- The extra starches you take in and the other foods that are converted into starches are stored in your thigh muscles and buttocks.
- When you sit, your thighs bear the weight of the pregnant uterus. Your thigh muscles therefore need exercise in pregnancy to firm and tone the muscles and keep them fit.

Preparing for labour

Depending on the position you decide to adopt, the thigh muscles play a very active role. It is important to prime the thighs in preparation for labour.

- Hold onto a table or firm chair and stand astride. Move down slowly with your back straight until you sit on your heels.
- Rest in that position for a minute then lift yourself up slowly until you are in a standing position. Repeat five times.

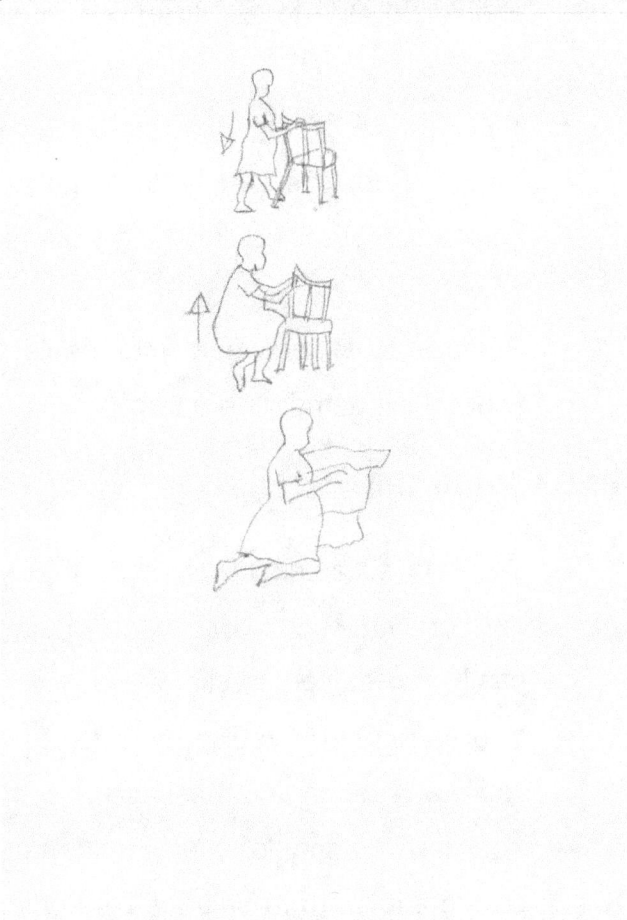

- You can work through this exercise together with your partner as your support as you hold hands and push yourself down then pull yourself up. You should be able to feel the thigh muscles contract.

- You can sit on the floor cross legged. Your partner sits astride and places his ankles on your knees pushing your knees down

- Practice to sit between your heels with your thighs astride like a frog.

BACK MASSAGE

- You can sit astride a chair so that your partner can kneel beside the chair and easily access your back.

- You can lean on your partner **(hug)** who can easily reach and massage your back. Your partner should stand astride or with one foot forward to balance his body and be able to support you especially if you should use this position while in labour where contractions may cause you to move uncontrollably.

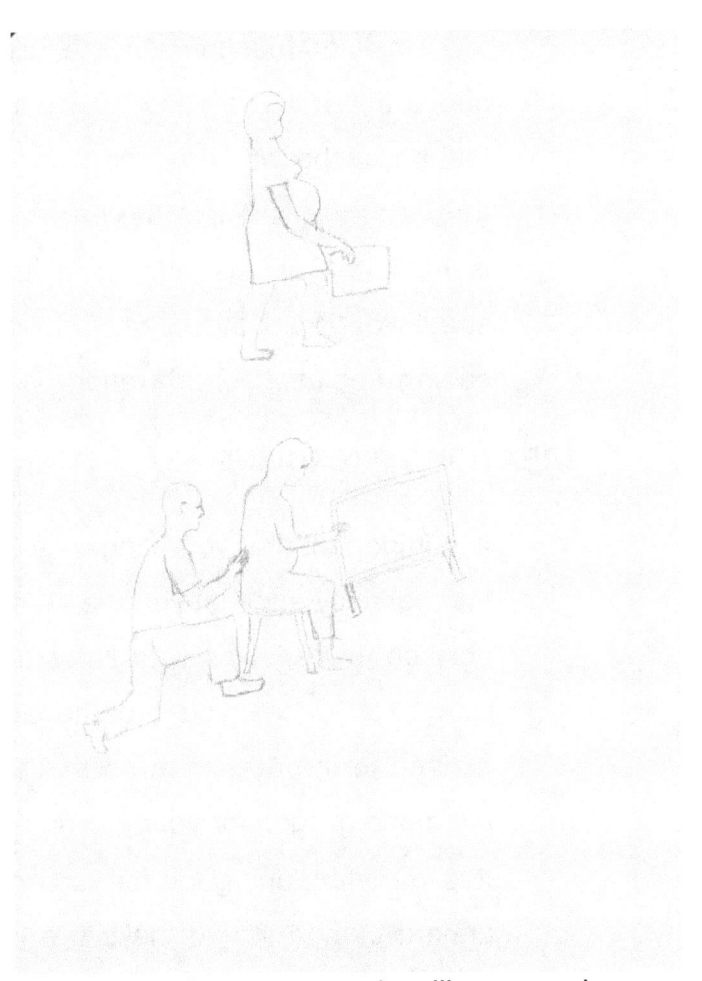

- You can throw several pillows and cushions on the floor and lean against them facing one side sitting on your heels with your legs astride. Your partner can sit on the side or kneel behind massaging

25

the small of the back or the area just above the buttocks gently. This is where the backache of late pregnancy is felt most and this is where the pain in labour is most felt as the abdominal muscles stretch out from this area. This position can also be used for relaxation.

BREATHING EXERCISES

- It is important that your lungs are healthy in pregnancy and that you are always in a position that enables your lungs to fill up with fresh air as you breathe and can expand to the maximum so that there is adequate oxygen for your growing baby.
- It is important and good for you and your unborn baby that you make it a habit to take early morning walks and walks in open air to enjoy fresh air.
- Around twenty-eight weeks you should engage in focused breathing exercises in preparation for labour.

- Take a deep breath through the nose and fill up your lungs then slowly breathe out through the mouth. Repeat the breaths three times in a minute. Continue to practice until you can repeat the breathing three times in five minutes.

Breathing during labour

When you feel the contraction come, you should get ready to breathe as the pain of the contraction begins.

- Breathe in and out while the heat of the contraction is still on, as the contraction wears off, relax. If you can take a nap go ahead and enjoy a nap in between the contractions.

Importance of breathing in labour

- As your muscles contract in labour they use up oxygen. Deep breaths supply your muscles with more oxygen.
- The pain of labour makes you restless and breathless. You need to take in large amounts of fresh air to supply your body with oxygen.
- The contractions squeeze the baby as they push the baby through the birth canal. As your baby is squeezed and pushed, he becomes breathless. When you breathe, you supply your baby with fresh oxygen to help him go through the stress of labour.
- Breathing relieves pain in labour through the increase of oxygen to muscles which reduces the 'cramp-like feeling' caused by the contractions.
- Breathing in labour reduces anxiety as it keeps you busy

Breathing during delivery of the baby

- Breathing is used to enable gentle delivery of baby and prevention of injury to the baby's head and the birth canal.
- Towards the end of labour health personnel will ask you to pant like a tired dog. These are shallow breaths that prevent you from rushing to push the baby out and enable the baby to slowly negotiate his way out without causing tears and bruises to the birth canal.

THE PELVIS

- The pelvis is made up of three bones. The two bones on the sides flare out at the top to form a dish like basin that forms the hip.
- The side bones meet in front to form the pubic bone. This joint is a soft cartilage joint that is covered by fat on which pubic hair grows.

- At the back the two pelvic bones are attached to the lower part of the spine.
- The lower part of the spine is made up of four bones that are fused to make one bone. These two joints are fixed and firm.
- The end of the spine ends as a sharp flexible bone that curls inwards between the buttocks like a little tail when you sit.
- The lower part of the pelvic bones flares out on the sides and the body rests on them when you sit.
- The pelvic bones are covered by ligaments and muscle that support them providing stability and helping to keep you in a good posture.
- The pelvic bones cushioned by ligaments and muscle form a protective basin that holds your bladder, womb and bowel.
- Pregnancy hormones soften your ligaments and your joints. The result of this softening of tissues is that you can

experience aches and pains especially in your back and your pelvic bones. The weight of the growing baby on the pelvic ligaments causes further aches and pains.

- Exercise in pregnancy helps to ease some of this discomfort around your pelvis by shifting the weight and easing pressure on certain joints.

PELVIC FLOOR MUSCLE EXERCISES

- During pregnancy, the flow of hormones in large quantities softens your smooth muscles. The pelvic floor muscles that form a corset below the pelvic bones and hold the pelvic contents in place are softened and relaxed by the pregnancy hormones.

- It is important to tone the pelvic floor muscles throughout pregnancy and keep them in shape.

- Loss of tone of pelvic floor muscles may be noticed by failure to hold urine which may dribble when laughing or coughing.
- Toning pelvic floor muscles is an exercise that can be done anywhere anytime and does not need preparation. It does not disturb your work or any routine of yours.

You can tone pelvic floor muscles wherever you are as follows:

- Pretend that your bladder is full and you have an urge to empty it but you cannot find a toilet. You pinch your muscles tight down below without squeezing your buttocks or moving your legs together and pull the muscles in for a count of three and relax the muscles.
- Repeat this exercise up to a count of ten whenever you can remember. This is a lifetime exercise for the woman!
- Continue this exercise throughout pregnancy. Try this exercise when having

sex; it enhances your partner's and your sexual enjoyment!

EXERCISE AFTER DELIVERY

After delivery of the baby

It is best to gradually take exercises to a higher level to tone up the muscles weakened by the effect of pregnancy hormones.

- The abdominal muscles stretched in pregnancy need to regain their tone.
- The extra weight gained due to cravings in pregnancy must burn up in order for a woman to regain shape.
- Post delivery, after engaging in more demanding exercises, you sleep well, and wake up refreshed and with renewed energy.

- Post delivery you need to eat well.

- **Exercise improves appetite** post delivery as you burn up stored energy, the body demands for food increase, the appetite improves.

- You need good nutrition that contains protein for repair of tissues worn out or bruised during pregnancy and labour. You need a diet rich in vitamins, minerals such as iron, calcium to improve lowered levels of blood components during pregnancy and labour.

- You need energy to breastfeed and carry out your motherhood chores.

When is the best time to exercise?

- Exercises are most effective and enjoyable if done first thing in the morning.

- Exercise done first thing in the morning is refreshing as the lungs fill with fresh cool air before the air is polluted by suit and smog from domestic, industrial and vehicle fumes.

- You are advised to exercise for a short period until you feel stronger and your body adjusts to the workout. Gradually increase the time spent exercising and vary the types of exercises.

- If however you feel very tired or your health is not very good, you need to slow down.

- Exercises are best done before a heavy meal. Your heart cannot cope with digesting a heavy meal as well as coping with exercise!

- You should do your exercises first, have a leisurely shower or bath which is also good at toning muscles, clearing away body wastes and refreshing you before you settle down to a meal.

- It is best to start with simple exercises and gradually increase the variety of your exercise until you feel strong enough to join local joggers in your area or go to the local gym and to the 'Keep Fit' group exercises

- Whether exercises are during pregnancy or post delivery, your partner can join in and enjoy the advantages of exercise. You feel supported and encouraged if your partner teams up with you.

- Pretend that your soggy tampon is about to drop or that you have a runny tummy but the toilet is a distance away. Pull the muscles in as if to keep the tampon in and to prevent the bowel from opening.

- Start exercising soon after delivery to tone the loose pelvic floor muscles.

- After the muscle relaxation caused by the pregnancy hormones, the stretch caused by the weight of the baby in late pregnancy and the stretch during delivery, your pelvic floor muscles need serious attention and toning up.

- Continue with the movements of the pelvic floor muscles as before but this time around you must pull in and hold for a count up to five, exercise more frequently and also assess how good your efforts are.

This is how you assess the tone of your pelvic floor muscles:

- Immediately after delivery, your muscles are very loose. Try this exercise as you take a bath and you will notice that your birth canal is wide open. Stick your index finger into your birth canal and pull your pelvic muscle in as you bath. You may not feel the grip of your muscles on the finger. Continue the exercise until your birth canal muscles can grip your index finger as you exercise. That is the first stage of toning up your muscles.

- Continue toning up your muscles until the muscles can grip your small finger! This is the second stage of pelvic floor muscle toning.

- The final stage is stopping the urine flow as you are half way emptying the bladder. You should be able to hold urine for a while then continue to empty the remaining amount. When you reach this stage, you must continue to exercise throughout your lifetime to maintain this pelvic floor muscle tone.

What happens if pelvic floor muscles remain loose?

- **Loose pelvic floor muscles can cause urine leaks and dribbles meaning you will always need a pad to receive the dribble.

- You are likely to always smell of urine, a very uncomfortable situation.

- Your pelvic organs can slip out through the loose muscles as you cough, sneeze, lift a heavy object or push a bowel motion. This is called a prolapsed of pelvic organs!

- **One can have a uterine prolapse, a rectal prolapse or a bladder prolapse!**
- A pelvic organ prolapse is a serious condition that is uncomfortable and embarrassing to live with.
- Organ prolapsed requires surgery to correct it.
- Avoid organ prolapse by simply following the above exercises!

TONING ABDOMINAL MUSCLES

- The abdominal muscles are attached to the sides of the chest, the back, and along the centre of the abdomen and the pelvis in front.
- During pregnancy the abdominal muscles must stretch forward to accommodate the growing womb.

- The muscles also pull on the back, changing the body structure and increasing the chances of a backache.
- After delivery abdominal muscles remain loose, bulky and flabby until you do something positive to tone them.

Do not tie a tight cloth around your abdomen as this does not tone your muscles but may interfere with good blood circulation which is needed for your body to heal.

Toning Abdominal muscles post delivery can be done this way:

- Start with simple deep breathing in and out pulling in the abdominal muscles as you breathe in.
- Deep breathing post delivery helps to expel blood from the womb.
- Deep breathing expands the lungs preventing lung complications especially **hypostatic pneumonia.**

- Lie down flat on your back with legs together and stretched. Stretch your arms above your head. Breathe in pulling in your abdominal muscles as you further stretch your arms and legs as far as possible. Repeat five to ten times.
- Put your hands on your side. Bend the left leg and put the foot of the bent leg flat on the floor.

  Keeping your right leg straight, lift it up as high as possible towards your tummy and put it down. Repeat ten times. Repeat these movements with your left leg while bending your right leg. This exercise tones your back, your buttocks, your thighs and your pelvic floor muscles.
- Lie flat on the floor. Bend one knee and pull it up over your abdomen as far as you can go. Repeat ten times with each leg. This exercise firms your thighs, your abdominal muscles and pelvic floor muscles.

- Sit up with legs stretched out and astride. Stretch your arms outwards. Tuck your tummy in as you stretch the right arm across to reach for your toes of the left foot ten times. Do the same with the left arm touching the toes on your right foot.

- Go on your fours with knees and arms apart. Breathe in pulling in your abdominal muscles stretching out your shoulders like an angry cat then breathe out repeatedly for five to ten times.

- Stand up with your feet astride. Swing your hands from side to side ten times to each side. This movement tightens the rings of muscles that look like flat tyres under your arms and upper abdomen.

Thigh muscles must be firmed so that they reduce in size and lose flabbiness.

- Stand up astride left hand on the hip, right hand stretched out. Stretch out the left leg in kicking movement as high as possible to reach out on the fingers of the stretched hand ten times then change to the right leg.

This exercise tones your back, your abdominal muscles, and your pelvic floor muscles and improves circulation in your legs reducing swelling in your legs.

- Bend your left knee to meet your bent right elbow in kicking movements ten times then do the same with the right leg.

- Stand up behind a chair and rest your arms on the back of the chair with your legs as wide apart as possible. Bend your knees slowly as you move your trunk downwards keeping your back straight. Hold your body in that position and feel your thigh muscles tighten up. Slowly pull yourself up and repeat movements up to five times.

- When you feel strong and able to withstand the programmed rhythmic exercises you can join the local 'Keep Fit Group'.

- Remember to keep fit you must eat a balanced diet. Weight gain is gradual so is weight loss.

Please note: **Do not go on crush programmes to lose weight. **

- Crush diets are unhealthy for your heart.
- Crush diets cause imbalance of essential food elements in your body system and may lead to such conditions like anaemia, eating disorders, and ulcers.
- You need a good diet to recover from effects of pregnancy and labour. You need a good diet everyday! Your everyday responsibilities require that you are strong. If you are a breast feeding mother you must have adequate milk for your baby.

EXERCISES FOR MATURE PEOPLE

Mature people need to exercise to keep blood flowing smoothly, prevent clots, varicose veins and swelling of feet. Mature people need to exercise to prevent stiffness of joints and to improve mobility.

It is best to exercise every part of the body where possible. You can start with any part of the body as follows:

Sit in a straight firm chair to prevent staggering and falls which may further reduce your mobility.

The head

Move your head from side to side five times.

Fill your cheeks with air and slowly blow out five times.

Move your face muscles slowly from side to side five times

Close your eyes tightly and open five times. These exercises prevent sagging of face muscles improve the tone of face muscles especially where one is recovering from facial paralysis and make you look youthful!

The chest

It is important that your heart and lungs are kept healthy. These two organs are vital organs to life. You need healthy lungs that can take in as much air as possible when you breathe in. Your heart needs fresh blood with lots of oxygen for it to pump blood well.

- Take a deep breath through the nose and slowly breathe out. Repeat five to ten times.

Arms

Keep your arms mobile and active.

- When you walk swing your arms to keep the joints flexible.
- While sitting in the chair, raise your arms as high as you can.
- Swing your arms from side to side five times
- Wave your hands from side to side (Mexican wave)

Enjoy your exercises!

References

Barlow,J; Coren,E. Parent-training programmes for improving maternal psychosocial health. PMID. *Cochrane Data Base System* Rev. 2004; (I) 4

Belloc, N. B; Breslow, L. Relationship of physical health status and health practices, *Preventive Medicine*,1972;9: 409-421

Balaskas, J.. *Active Birth. Unwin Paperbacks*, 1989. London.

Daley, A; Jolly, K; Macarthur, C.) The effectiveness of exercise in the management of postnatal depression: systematic review and meta-analysis. *Family Practitioner,* 2009; (3): 35-41

Lee, C. (1998). *Women's Health: Psychological and Social Perspectives.* California: Sage Publications.

www.ingramcontent.com/pod-product-compliance
Lightning Source LLC
Chambersburg PA
CBHW070341290526
45791CB00003B/1418